Per & Carina Nyberg

The Hallux Valgus Cure

A Simple And Natural Method for Pain-Free Feet

Expendo Publishing

Disclaimer

The material contained in this book is for informational purposes only. The author and anyone else affiliated with the creation or distribution of this book may NOT be held liable for damages of any kind whatsoever allegedly caused or resulting from any such claimed reliance. Before using these exercises, it is recommended that you consult with your physician for authorization and clearance. It is always recommended to consult with a physician before beginning any new exercise or nutritional program. If you have any problems with your health, you should seek clearance from a qualified medical professional. The information contained herein is not intended to, and never should, substitute for the necessity of seeking the advice of a qualified medical professional.

The Hallux Valgus Cure: A Simple and Natural Method for Pain-Free Feet

Published by Expendo Publishing
ISBN: 978-91-981693-2-4

Table of contents

1. Introduction

Despite the fact that we use our feet every day, and that they really act as a platform for our entire body, most of us seldom stop to think about how important our feet really are. If we did stop to think about it, we would see that our feet actually fulfill vital functions in most movements that we perform during an average day; from regular activities such as standing up or going for a short walk, to more demanding workouts. Our feet are built to endure quite a lot – in a normal jogging session, the load on the foot can be up to *four times* our own bodyweight.

It can seem a bit paradoxical considering our relatively high living standards, and all the modern comforts that many of us surround ourselves with in our society, but the fact is that an increasing number of people are suffering from painful and limiting feet disorders. Although the majority of us are born with functionally perfect feet, a multitude of different of foot related disorders can develop as we grow older. Only then do we start to understand how vitally important our feet really are for us, and the degree to which we depend on our feet to perform different activities in our daily lives. When our feet hurt, a simple walk to the mailbox can become a real torture.

So – what are the root causes of these painful foot disorders then? Well, there are obviously several factors in play here, but one of the main causes that many of us develop some form of chronic feet pain sooner or later is that the human foot is a very intricate construction, that really isn't adapted to the kind of terrain – mainly hard, flat surfaces – that we spend most of our time standing or walking around upon.

But often, we also aggravate the problem ourselves, mainly because of the following two factors:

- *Wrong shoes.* One could argue that wearing shoes at all is something that is unnatural for us human beings – not to mention narrow, high-heeled shoes. High-heeled shoes can actually increase the load on the anterior part of the foot with up to 75 %! Since our feet really aren't made to spend so much time in shoes, it shouldn't come as a surprise to us that this can lead to many different foot disorders. But even though the problem might manifest itself somewhere in the foot, the actual cause of the problem doesn't always emanate *from* the foot. This discussion is continued in chapter 4.

- *A physically inactive lifestyle* can also contribute to different foot-related conditions. This is partly because our feet need a certain amount of training to function optimally, but also because physical inactivity negatively affects several functions – such as blood circulation – within the whole body.

2. About Hallux Valgus

Hallux Valgus is a foot-related condition where the joint of the big toe becomes deformed and tilts outward, so the big toe itself tilts inwards, towards the other toes (*hallux* means big toe and *valgus* means bent or angled). The rest of the toes usually become a bit crowded, as a result of the inward angle of the big toe. Furthermore, as a result of the tilted toe joint, Hallux Valgus also leads to the forming of a bunion at the side of the joint of big toe. The picture illustrates how the early phase of a Hallux Valgus-condition can look – as we can see, the bunion at the side of the big toe is more prominent on the right foot than on the left.

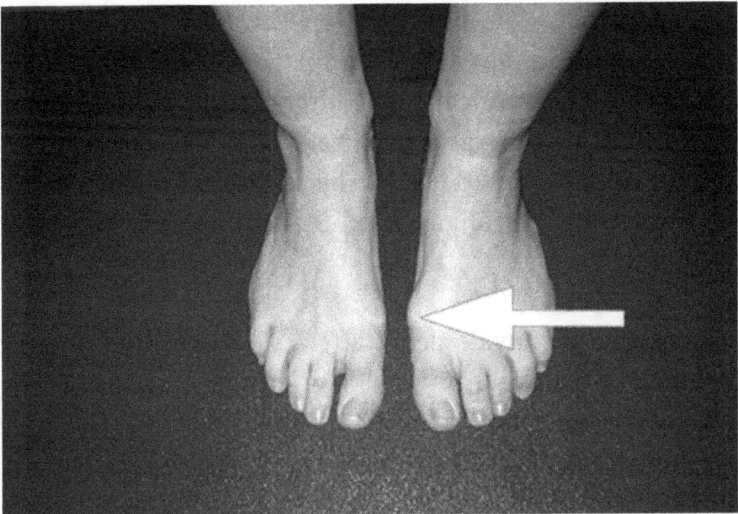

Picture 2.1: The early phase of Hallux Valgus.

Usually, this bunion becomes quite sore, which leads to more pain and fatigue in the forefoot area. With time, the bunion can also become inflamed, leading to even more pain and discomfort in this area.

As the condition develops and becomes worse, this usually leads to a number of practical problems, such as finding shoes that doesn't further aggravate the pain. In reality, many people experience more or less daily discomfort, even when using "foot-friendly" shoes with plenty of room in the front. Scientific studies state that sooner or later, Hallux Valgus afflicts approximately 25 % of the population. If the discomfort is classified as minor to medium, some kind of orthopedic aid is often recommended; such as specially designed shoes, different shoe pads, or toe splints that temporarily reduce the pain and/or pull the big toe back in the opposite direction.

If the condition develops even further, surgery is usually necessary. The surgical procedure is performed with the aid of local or general anaesthesia, and can take up to 40 minutes. To turn the big toe back into its normal position, the joint is realigned and fixated with wires, screws or plates.

The period of convalescence after a Hallux Vallux surgery will of course differ, but 6-8 weeks is not unusual. The forefoot is normally swollen for about 2-3 months after the surgery, but in some cases the swelling can actually remain for as long as a year after the procedure.

Relaterad foot conditions

As a result of the tilted big toe, Hallux Valgus can also lead to the development of a condition called *hammer toe*, where one or more of the remaining toes end up in a bent position, which often results in painful callosities on top of the toes and below the foot pad. To alleviate this condition, the general recommendation is to use shoes with plenty of room in the front, as well as some kind of arch support.

The development of hammer toe can, in turn, lead to the development of a *club-* or *claw* toe. In a hammer toe, the condition affects the innermost joint of the toe, but in a club toe it is the outermost joint that is affected. When all three joints in a toe becomes bent, this is called a claw toe. Furthermore, the same basic complex of problems that leads to hammer-, club-, and claw toes is also a contributing factor to a number of heel-related foot conditions, such as heel fissures and heel spurs.

What causes Hallux Valgus?

So far, the scientific research within the area has been unable to come up with a unequivocal answer to this seemingly simple question. Generally, the use of tight and narrow shoes are pointed out as the most likely suspect. Statistically, the majority of the people – approximately 80 % – that are afflicted by foot related disorders are women, and Hallux Valgus is unfortunately no exception to this rule; about 9 out of 10 that suffer from Hallux Valgus are women. This fact is another main reason that tight or high-heeled shoes are assigned most of the blame when it comes to the development of Hallux Valgus, although certain findings imply that this might not be the whole truth. It has actuallybeen discovered that Hallux Valgus also develops in populations that rarely wear shoes at all, so we obviously need to take other factors into account as well.

On the other hand, it is probably still likely that our choice of shoes plays a certain role in the development of Hallux Valgus, but maybe not to the extent – or even primarily – for the reasons we have suspected. This discussion is further elaborated upon in chapter 5.

3. Basic anatomy of the foot and the calf

To understand the logic behind the methods presented in this book, and why they actually work when it comes to preventing and treating Hallux Valgus, we first need to discuss some basic anatomy in relation to the foot and the calf. Let's start with *the foot*.

About the foot

The human foot is an extremely intricate construction, which consists of many different joints, muscles, ligaments, and nerve endings. One human foot consists of 26-28 different bones (yes, it can differ from one individual to another) and over 200 muscles, tendons and ligaments. Actually, 25 % of all the bones in the human body are located in our feet. Furthermore, our feet contain approximately 70 000 nerve endings and more than 60 different joints, so maybe it shouldn't come as much of a surprise to us that many of us sooner or later are afflicted by some kind of painful foot condition.

In relation to the purpose of this book, the part of the foot called the *Plantar Fascia* plays an important role. The Plantar Fascia is a thick layer of fibrous, connective tissue, and its main purpose is to support the arch of the foot, thereby helping the body to cushion the shock when we walk, jump or run.

For example, the Plantar Fascia is often mentioned in connection with heel spurs, but in this book we are more interested in directing our focus towards the front part of the foot, since this connective tissue also acts as a kind of link between our toes and our heel. In practice, this means that a rigid and shortened Plantar Fascia also potentially affects what goes on with our toes.

We seldom give this much thought, but our toes are actually much more important to us than we usually give them credit for, since they act to help us maintain balance when we stand and stabilize the forward movement when we walk or run. If you don't believe this statement, simply try to walk quickly forward while pointing your toes upwards, and you will find that your walk will feel very unnatural and rigid.

The big toe is particularily important in relation to the Plantar Fascia and the stabilization of the foot arch. The stabilizing function of our toes becomes even more apparent in activities that challenges our balance, such as ice-skating.

In reality, our feet are designed in almost the same way as our hands, even if our hands and our feet look quite different from each other today. Another aspect in relation to our toes is that we actually can use them to "grab" the ground when we stand, walk, or even run. The use of shoes makes this feature less apparent, but when our feet are bare the toes can help stabilizing the entire body by naturally performing a gripping action against the surface below us. This balance- and stability aspect is most apparent when performing one-legged movements, so feel free to stand on one leg for a while to see if you can feel the increased activation of the toes.

About the calf

The biggest muscle on the lower leg is generally referred to as the *three-headed calf muscle*. At the bottom, the calf muscle is connected to the Achilles tendon, close to the heel bone.

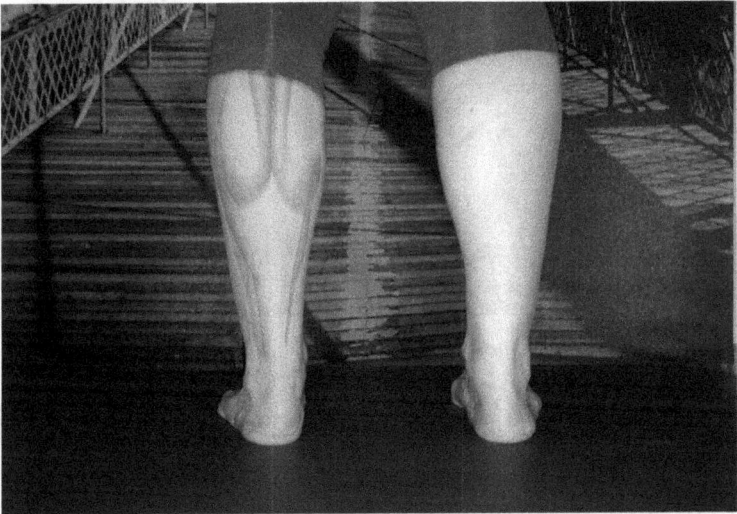

Picture 3.1: The three-headed calf muscle.

There are quite a few muscles and tendons in connection with the lower leg, but for our purposes, the following muscles and tendons are probably the most important ones:

- **Gastrocnemius**
- **Soleus**
- **Peroneus Longus**
- **Tibialis Anterior**
- **The Achilles tendon**

Gastrocnemius

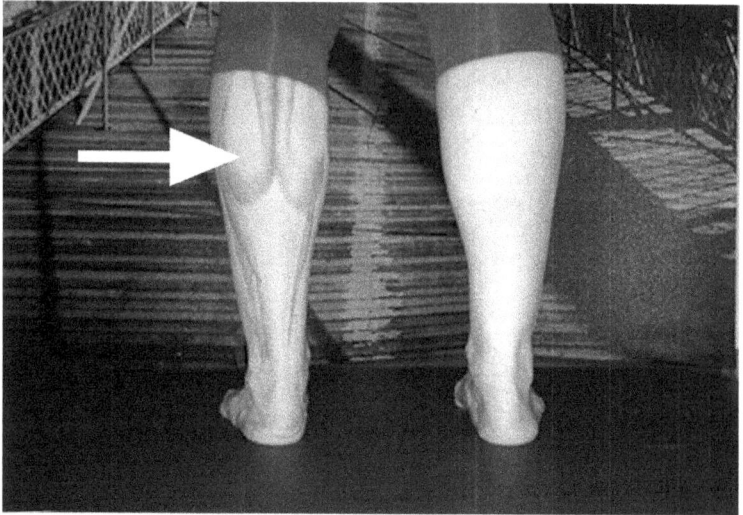

Picture 3.2: Gastrocnemius.

Gastrocnemius is generally referred to as the outer calf muscle, and it is situated on the back of the lower leg, as illustrated by the picture. Gastrocnemius connects downwards to the heel – which, in turn, is connected to the Plantar Fascia – and upwards on both sides of the thigh bone, just above the knee.

This means that a rigid and shortened calf muscle may affect both the Plantar Fascia and the toes. Gastrocnemius is activated when we walk, run or jump.

Soleus

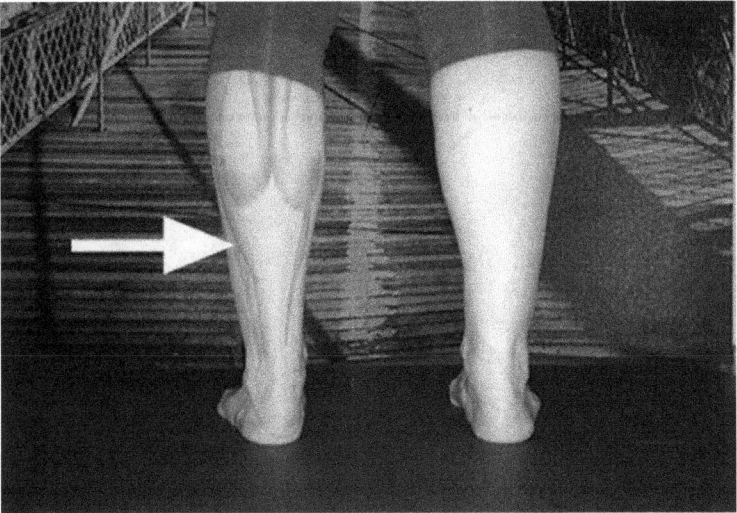

Picture 3.3: Soleus.

Soleus is an inner, deeply situated part of the calf muscle. Soleus originates from the upper part of the tibia (also known as the shinbone) and the fibula, and connects downwards to the Achilles tendon and the heel bone. Its main function is to extend the foot at the ankle joint. Soleus helps us maintain balance, and is activated when we are in a standing position.

Peroneus Longus

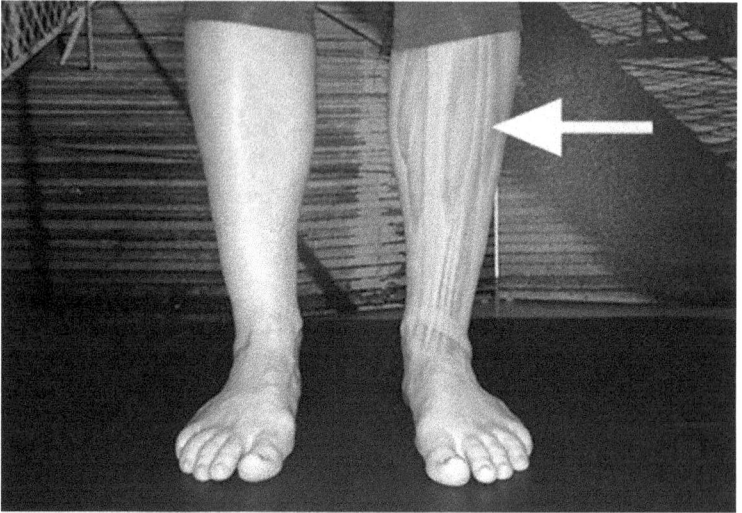

Picture 3.4: Peroneus Longus.

Peroneus Longus is a muscle that is located on the outside of the calf, and its main function is to extend and move the foot outwards. Peroneus Longus also helps us maintaining our balance, especially in various one-legged movements.

Tibialis Anterior

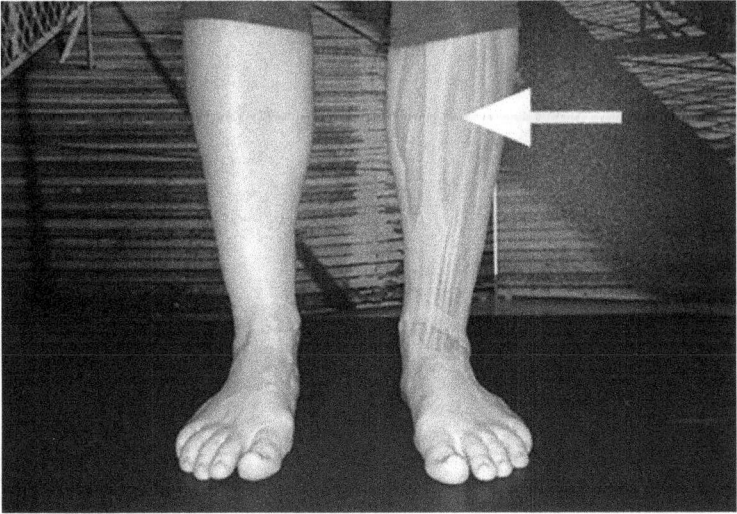

Picture 3.5: Tibialis Anterior.

Tibialis Anterior extends over the tibia, and the word anterior indicates that it is situated in front of the tibia. The main function of Tibialis Anterior is to rotate the foot inwards and to pull it upwards. Just like many other calf muscles, Tibialis Anterior helps with stability when we walk or run.

The Achilles tendon

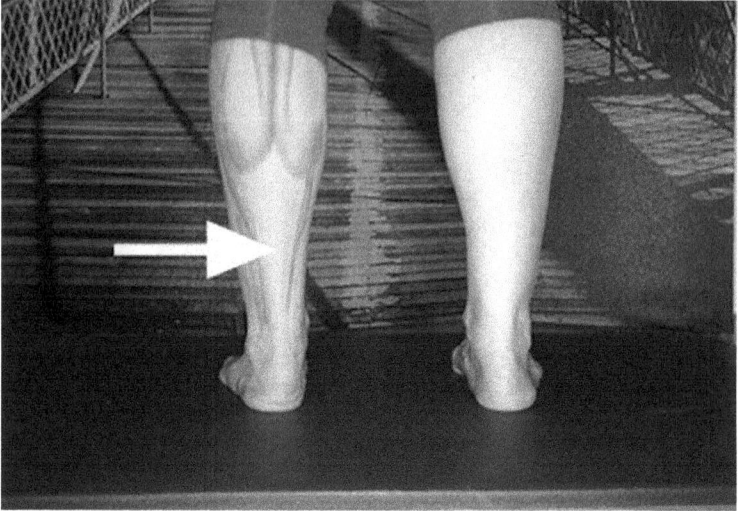

Picture 3.6: The Achilles tendon.

The Achilles tendon is in fact the strongest and thickest tendon in the entire body. It is subjected on a daily basis to a lot of stress, especially when we run or jump. A lot of people – especially among avid runners – develop more or less chronic pain in the Achilles tendon, most likely due to too much physical stress.

It is quite common to hear about inflammation in connection with the pain related to the Achilles tendon, but the fact is that this pain not always can be attributed to inflammatory changes. Even though numerous studies have been performed on the subject, we still can't say with absolute certainty why we develop chronic pain in the Achilles tendon.

4. Hallux Valgus – an alternative treatment

When it comes to traditional treatment of the Hallux Valgus-condition, a multitude of more or less expensive orthopedic aids exist, many of them designed to pull the big toe back into its normal position. However, the main problem with these orthopedic aids is that none of them really addresses the root cause of the condition – instead, they focus primarily on the symptoms. Of course, this also means that the condition most likely will return as soon as we stop using the aid. Along similar lines of logic, a surgical procedure can be performed to realign the joint and thus – more or less temporary – get rid of the pain. Unfortunately, the condition will often gradually return even after a successful surgery, which clearly indicates that the root cause of the condition hasn't been addressed.

Like so many other discoveries, the treatment that is advocated in this book was discovered more or less by coincidence. Actually, the purpose of the treatment was originally to alleviate a knee-related condition by treating adjacent tissue, by using some of the exercises that are described later in this book. However, one of the test subjects had also started to develop Hallux Valgus a couple of years before, and – to our surprise – the treatment also had a direct effect on this condition. To our surprise, the treatment had an almost immediate effect when it came to relieving the pain. As the treatment continued, the pain gradually disappeared completely. To us, this was an unexpected but very interesting result, since the scientific research within the field hasn't been able to deduce why we develop Hallux Valgus in the first place.

This discovery made us take a closer look at the traditional methods for treating Hallux Valgus. As we have discussed, the recommended treatment methods are focused on the specific area where the problem arises, which is the front of the foot. This becomes quite clear when we take a look at all the orthopedic aids that are available for pain relief; such as wider shoes, toe splints and shoe pads. However, our discovery pointed us in the opposite direction and indicated that the root of the problem wasn't necessarily to be found in the foot itself. Even though our exercises were focused on the calf muscle rather than the foot, the result was still a gradual reduction of the foot-related pain. After having been able to try out the method on even more test subjects, we are convinced that this is related to the way our fascia and our muscles function and connect to each other. In this chapter, we will explain how and why our method works.

It is important to emphasize that this treatment is based upon methods that, from a general perspective, are both proven and established – even though these methods haven't been adapted for or used specifically to treat Hallux Valgus before. However, the specific exercises and methods that are advocated in this book are the results of our own deductions, based upon our direct experiences and observations during and after working with our test subjects. The actual exercises will be described in chapter 5, but it is important to first understand how and why these exercises really work. Therefore, we will start by explaining and discussing the following concepts:

- **Kinetic chains**
- **Self Myofascial Release**
- **The Fascia**
- **Stretching**

Kinetic chains

In the context of kinetic chains, we usually hear about the concepts of *open* and *closed* movement chains. However, in relation to this particular treatment method, these specific concepts are not something that we need to take into consideration. The basic idea of kinetic chains emanates from the perspective that different parts of our bodies cannot be isolated from each other when we perform various movements – and that a movement around a specific joint also affects the closest joints, above and below the joint in which the movement was initiated.

For instance, the position of the ankle when we walk or run can sometimes lead to knee-related issues, which in turn can result in hip-related issues. If the hip joint is in a faulty position, this can lead to various back-related problems – and so on, further up (or down) the kinetic chain.

In this book we are mainly interested in following a particular part of the kinetic chain the other way; from the lower leg and down via the heel, all the way to the toes.

Self Myofascial Release

The word myofascia is built up by two parts; *myo*, meaning muscle tissue and *fascia*, a connective tissue that can be found in a lot of different places inside our bodies. The words *self* and *release* indicates that this is a kind of treatment that we can perform ourselves, and that the treatment has a liberating or relaxing effect. In other words, *Self Myofascial Release* is a simple way to work through and release built-up stiffness and tension in both the fascia and the muscles by combining movement and pressure. The muscle tonus – meaning the tension in the muscle fibers when the muscle is in a resting state – is also reduced as a result of the SMR-treatment. In summary, the purpose of SMR is to increase our mobility by gradually increasing the quality of our muscles, fascia, ligaments and tendons.

The basis for the effectiveness of SMR-treatment is a principle called *autogenic inhibition*. The way autogenic inhibition works is related to the function of a proprioceptive sensory receptor called the *Golgi tendon organ*. This sensory receptor is weaved into the tendon, exactly at the transition point between the tendon and the muscle, and its purpose is to determine the load on the muscle/tendon in any given moment. When the level of tension in the muscle/tendon becomes too high, these receptors are pinched, which in turn makes the muscle automatically relax. This automatic relaxation reflex is actually a kind of defense mechanism, which protects the tendon from overstretching – which otherwise potentially could lead to a muscle tear. By using SMR, we can consciously and safely activate the mechanisms in the Golgi tendon organ that makes the muscle relax – and when the muscle relaxes, it becomes softer and easier to massage, which helps to increase the effect of the continued SMR-treatment.

The role of the fascia

The *fascia* is a layer of thin, fibrous tissue that stretches all over our bodies – surrounding bones, organs and muscles – and its purpose is to hold together and stabilize different kinds of tissues and organs.

Considering how we made the discovery that resulted in the development of this specific method for treating Hallux Valgus, it is very interesting to note that the concept of connective tissue massage also was discovered by mere coincidence. What we today refer to as connetive tissue massage or connetive tissue therapy was discovered by the german physiotherapist *Elisabeth Dicke* back in the 1930's. Dicke was suffering from a quite serious blood circulation disorder in one of her legs, and the doctors told her that there was noting they could do – her leg would have to be amputated. While she was waiting for surgery, she desperately started to massage her lower back, and noticed how the blood circulation in her leg slowly but gradually improved. Eventually, she made a complete recovery.

Of course, today we know a lot more about the fascia, even if there still are aspects that we don't understand completely in relation to this tissue. What we do know is that the fascia is an important component in the so-called *fascial muscle chains*. Since we discussed kinetic chains earlier in this chapter, it might be a good idea to clarify the difference between kinetic chains and fascial muscle chains.

Generally speaking, both fascial muscle chains and kinetic chains are ways to describe how different structures in our bodies are connected to and influence each other, but from a slightly different perspective. When we talk about kinetic chains, we mainly focus on the way movement in a specific joint affects other, adjacent joints. Rather than focusing on the movement in a particular joint, the concept of fascial muscle chains aims to describe how the fascia and the muscle tissue are connected to and affect each other. Fascial muscle chains are sometimes compared to "anatomy trains", where the initiating muscle works almost as a locomotive, pulling a number of train wagons behind itself – which actually is a quite good comparison.

There are a number of different muscle chains – the *posterior*, *anterior* and *diagonal* chains, for instance – that run all over our bodies. However, we don't need to go into any detail when it comes to these muscle chains – for our purposes, we only need to understand that different structures in our bodies are connected in a multitude of ways. The fascia plays an important part when it comes to tying our muscles, ligament and joint together into these chains.

The muscle chains that we will focus on here are the anterior and the posterior muscle chains. Most likely, the posterior muscle chain is particularily interesting in relation to Hallux Valgus, since this muscle chain starts at the bottom of the foot, just behind the toes, and extends through the back of the body and over the head – all the way to the eyebrows.

Stretching

If we take a closer look at what current research has to say about stretching, it quickly becomes apparent that this still is a somewhat controversial subject. Furthermore, there are several different types of stretching – like *static*, *dynamic* and *ballistic* stretching – which further contributes to the confusion. To sum it all up, the fact is that most studies in the field assert that stretching has no apparent effect on the length of a muscle – even though the occasional study claims the opposite. But – and this is important – this is not the same thing as saying that stretching has no effect at all. The majority of studies also show that stretching muscles results in increased mobility – even though the length of the muscle doesn't change. The reason for the increase in mobility has not been made clear yet, but one theory is that the central nervous system is affected in a way that allows an increased movement range in and around the actual muscle.

It is not always easy to know if a certain muscle is shortened or tight (or both), since both these states can be perceived in a very similar way. As described in an earlier chapter, the SMR-treatment works mainly by affecting the quality and the tonus of the muscle, by softening the muscle tissue, fascia and any existing scar tissue from old injuries – which makes these exercises a great preparation for stretching the muscle.

The type of stretching that is described in this book is what we call *passive static stretching*. This type of stretching has produced very good results when it comes to increasing the *plasticity*, i. e. the *mobility*, in the musculature. This is exactly what we want to achieve by using the simple stretches outlined in this book; to quickly and permanently increase the mobility of the calf muscle. Increased mobility in and around muscles and joints also decreases the risk for muscle ruptures, as well as tendon injuries. However, it is important to understand that stretching performed in the wrong way can have the opposite effect, which is the reason that we perform the SMR-exercises *first* and then go on to stretch the already softened tissue.

5. Exercises

The exercises are simple to perform and don't require much equipment. You only need the following things:

- **2-3 tennis balls**
- **A small, soft textile bag (alternatively, a sock can also be used)**

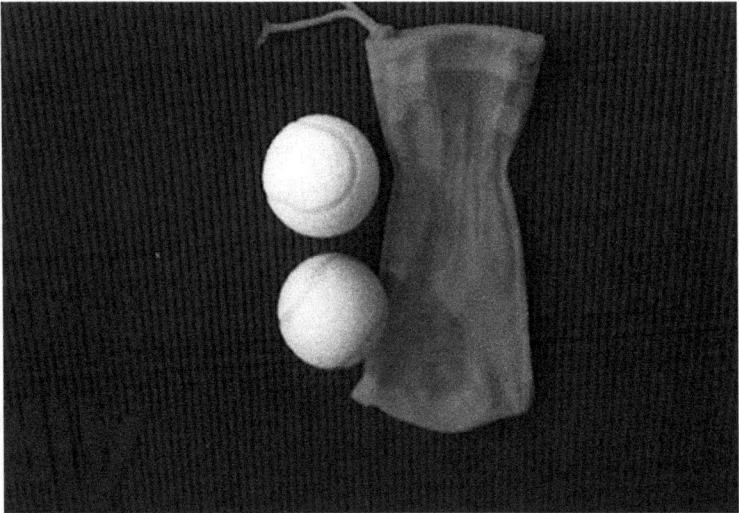

Picture 5.1: Two tennis balls and a small bag.

- **A string or a rubber band to seal the bag**
- **A chair or a similar, flat surface of approximately the same height**

As was discussed in chapter 4, these exercises combines Self Myofascial Release and passive static stretching. For best results, it is recommended that the exercises should be performed at least every other day, especially in the beginning of the treatment. After approximately 2-3 weeks, the frequency can be reduced to two times per week, assuming that the pain in connection to the toe joint has diminished. It is difficult to say exactly how long this will take, since it largely depends on the severity of the Hallux Valgus-condition. Thus, the time it takes to achieve the desired effect of the treatment will always differ somewhat from one individual to another.

Even though the exercises themselves aren't very physically demanding, it is important to to be able to move freely, so we recommend using comfortable clothes with a loose fit. Since the SMR-treatment has an essential massaging effect on the tissue, shorts or relatively short tights are recommended. To get the most out if the SMR-exercises, the calves should be bare.

Basic guidelines

- Place the tennis balls next to each other in the bag/ sock and seal the bag, so that the balls are kept in place, as the picture shows.

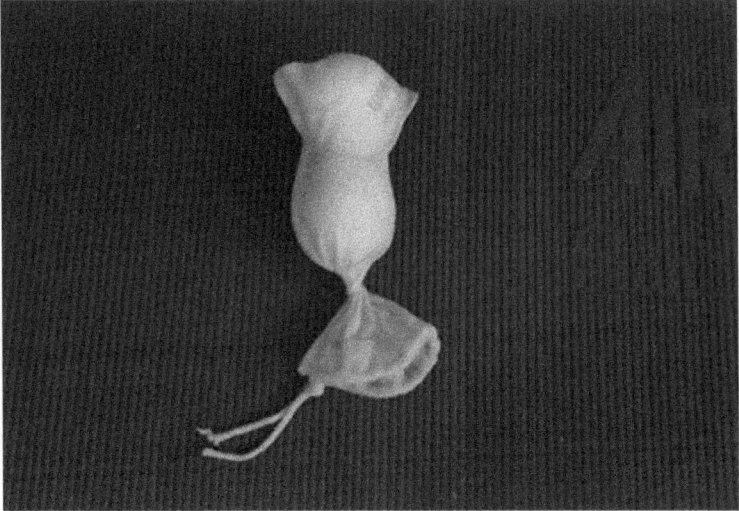

Picture 5.2: The tennis balls placed in the bag.

- Adjust the pressure depending on the level of discomfort. If it is very painful, apply a little less pressure, and if you don't feel any discomfort at all, you most likely need to gradually increase the amount of pressure. On a scale from 1 to 10 the perceived level of discomfort should not be higher than 7.

- When performing the exercises, try to stay relaxed and breathe calmly.

- Perform every exercise continuously for approximately 1 minute, by slowly moving the leg back and forth on top of the balls. Take a short break for about 30-60 seconds before moving on to the next exercise.

- If any area hurts more than others during the SMR-exercises, this is often an indication that this area needs a little extra attention. Therefore, it is a good idea to focus on this particular spot for a while (but don't neglect the rest – the whole muscle should be treated).

- Always perform the SMR-exercises first, and the stretching afterwards, in the exact order that is outlined in this chapter.

- To increase the effect of the SMR-exercises, use lacrosse balls (or a similar type of harder balls) instead of the tennis balls. Be prepared that this can hurt a bit more, especially if your calf muscles are very tense.

- If you perform the exercises on both of your legs, finish all of the exercises on one leg before moving on to the other leg.

Exercise 1

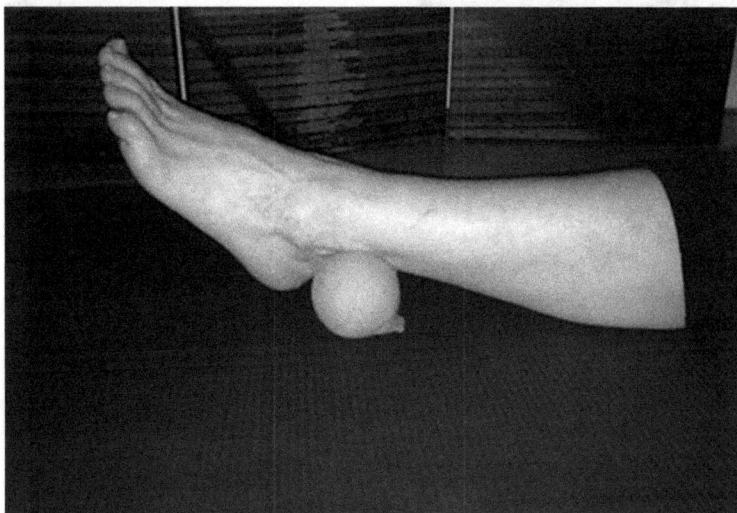

Picture 5.3: Exercise 1, step 1.

Place the leg so that the balls are positioned just above the heel, as the above picture shows. Next, move the leg slowly forward, so the calf "rolls" on top of the balls, while using the bodyweight to apply sufficient pressure.

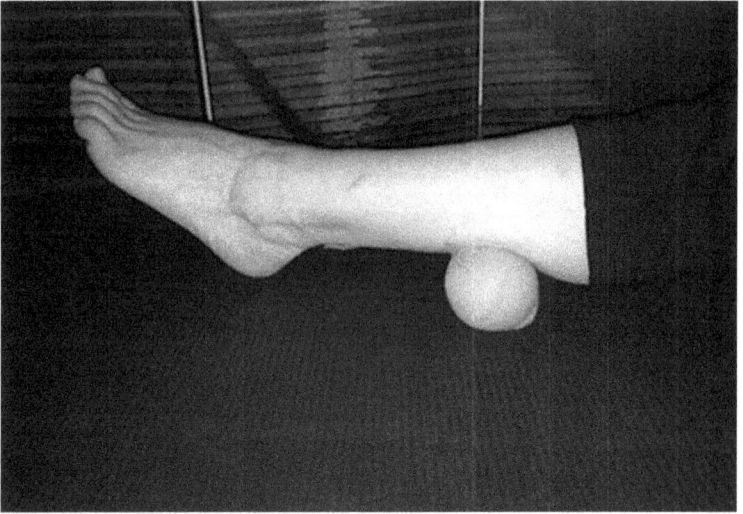

Picture 5.4: Exercise 1, step 2.

Continue to slowly move the leg forward, so the position of the balls moves further up the calf muscle. Try to maintain an even amount of pressure against the balls.

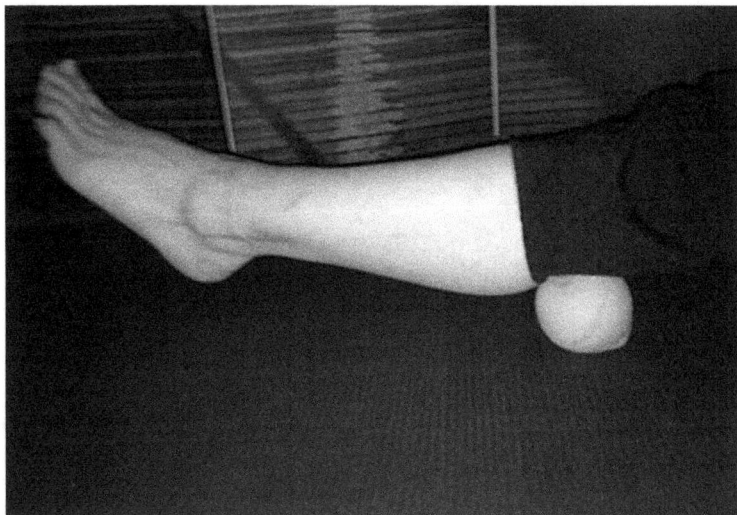

Picture 5.5: Exercise 1, step 3.

Keep moving the leg slowly forward, so the balls continue to roll upwards on the calf muscle. Stop just below the back of the knee and reverse the movement by starting to move the leg in the opposite direction.

Now, it is just a matter of moving the leg back and forth over the balls for at least 1 minute. Try to find a rhythm in the movement that allows you to move back and forth about 3-4 times during this time. It is not absolutely vital that you perform the exercise for exactly one minute, but it is a good rule of thumb. If you are unsure about the speed of the movement, it is always better to lower the tempo slightly.

Exercise 2

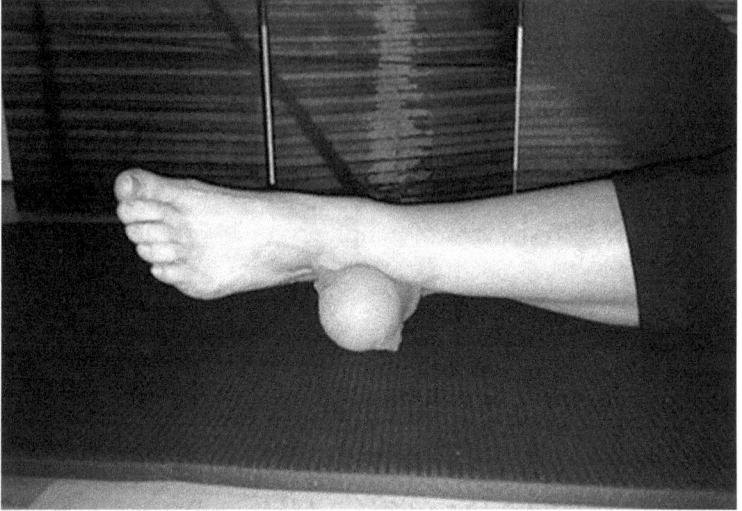

Picture 5.6: Exercise 2, step 1.

In exercise number 2, it is time to focus on the outer part of the calf muscle. Place the balls just above the external malleolus, as the picture shows. Next, slowly move the leg forward so the balls roll up on the outside of the calf muscle, in the same way as in exercise number 1.

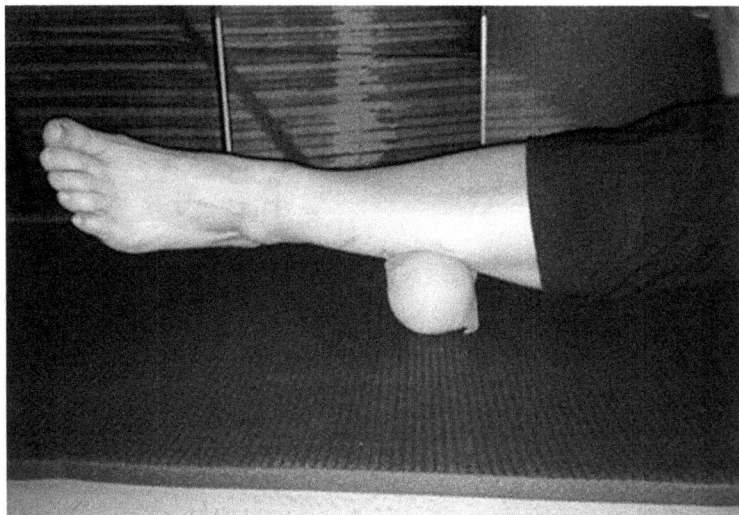

Picture 5.7: Exercise 2, step 2.

Continue to slowly move the leg forward, so the balls keep rolling upwards on the outside of the calf muscle.

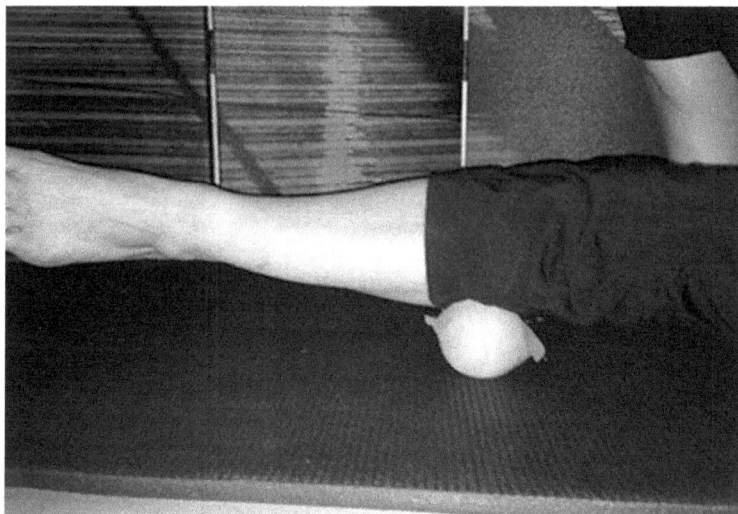

Picture 5.8: Exercise 2, step 3.

Just as before, keep moving the leg slowly forward, so the balls continue to roll upwards on the outside of the calf muscle. Stop just below the side of the knee joint and reverse the movement by starting to move the leg in the opposite direction.

Just as in exercise number 1, the movement should be performed slowly and continuously, back and forth. Perform the movement for at least 1 minute, which equals approximately 3-4 turns.

Exercise 3

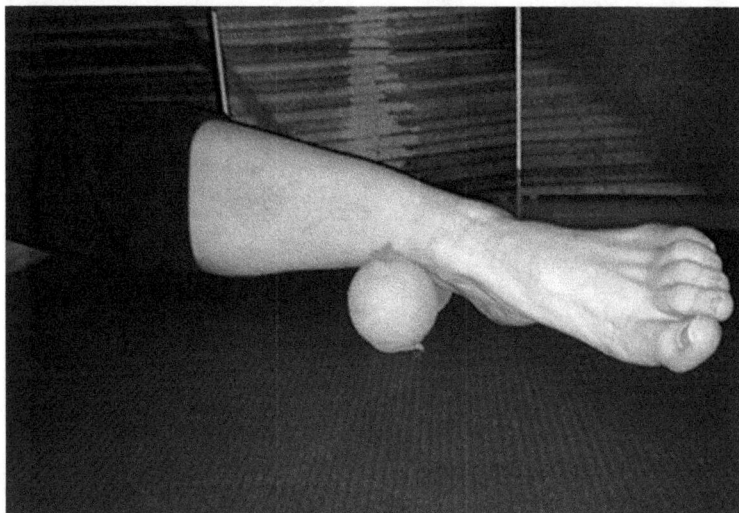

Picture 5.9: Exercise 3, step 1.

In exercise number 3, the time has come to focus on the inner side on the calf muscle. Place the bag with the balls just above the internal malleolus, as illustrated in the picture. Then, just as before, slowly move the leg forward so the balls roll up on the inner side of the calf muscle, in the same way as in exercises 1 and 2.

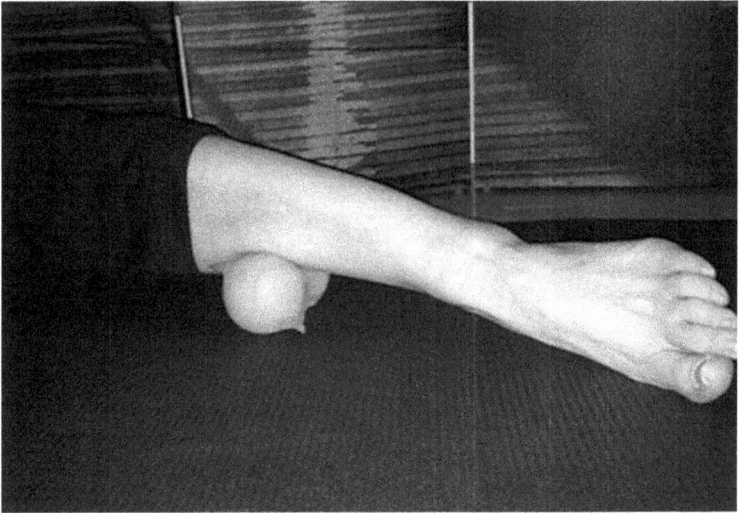

Picture 5.10: Exercise 3, step 2.

Continue to slowly move the leg forward, so the balls keep rolling upwards on the inner side of the calf muscle.

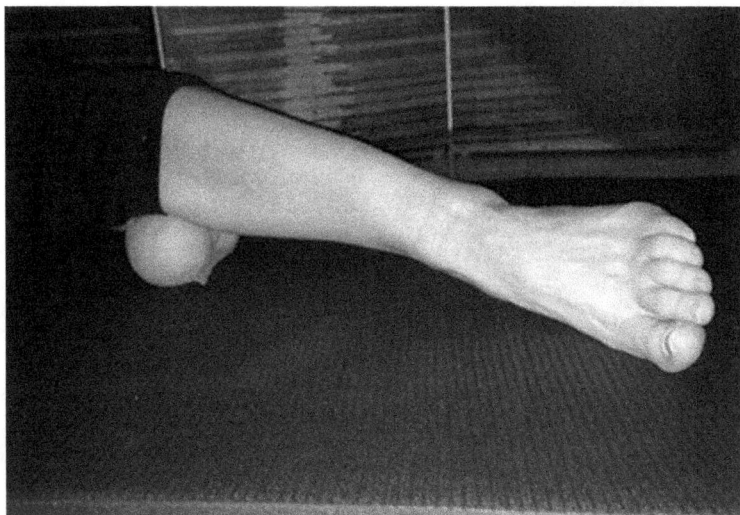

Picture 5.11: Exercise 3, step 3.

Keep moving the leg slowly forward, so the balls continue to roll upwards on the inner side of the calf muscle. Stop just below the side of the knee joint and reverse the movement by starting to move the leg in the opposite direction.

Like the other SMR-exercises, exercise number 3 should be performed continuously for at least 1 minute. Next, move on to exercise number 4.

Exercise 4

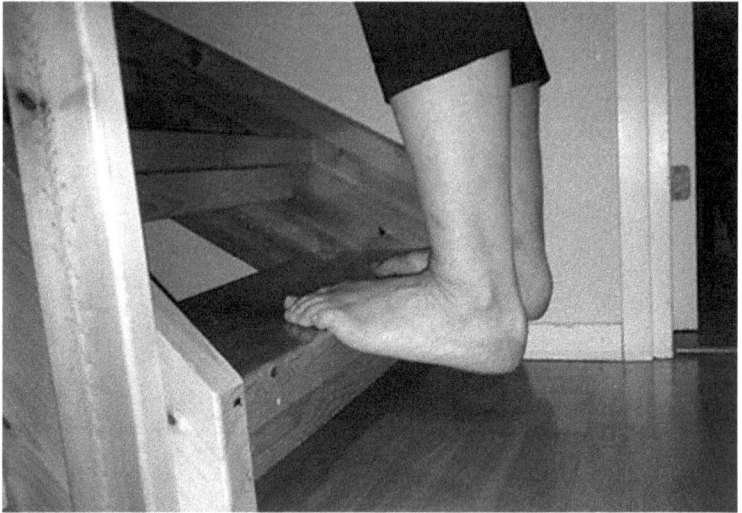

Picture 5.12: Exercise 4.

Since the purpose of the first 3 exercises has been to massage and soften the muscle and the fascia on the back of the lower leg, the next step is to stretch the softened muscle. This stretch is most easily performed by placing the front of the foot on an elevated surface, like a stair or a doorstep.

Then, just try to relax your calf muscle and let the heel "hang" over the ledge of the elevated surface. Hold this stretch for about 60 seconds. Take a short break (approximately 15-30 seconds) and do one more set of this stretch, in exactly the same way.

Exercise 5

In exercise number 5, the time has come to shift focus from the back of the lower leg to the front of the lower leg. This exercise can also be performed on the floor, but we recommend using a chair, as illustrated by the next picture.

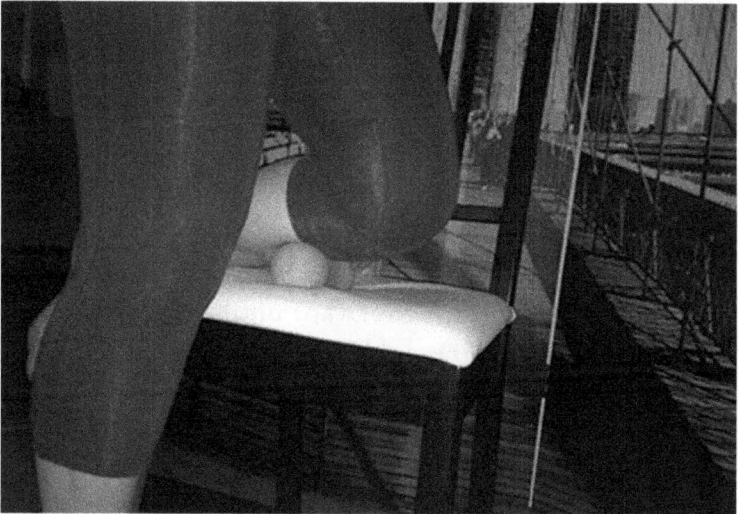

Picture 5.13: Exercise 5, step 1.

Place the bag containing the balls on the seat of the chair and position the front of the lower leg on top of the balls, just below the knee cap. Next, slowly move the leg forward, so that the balls roll downward, moving closer to the foot. If necessary, hold on to the back of the chair to help with balance.

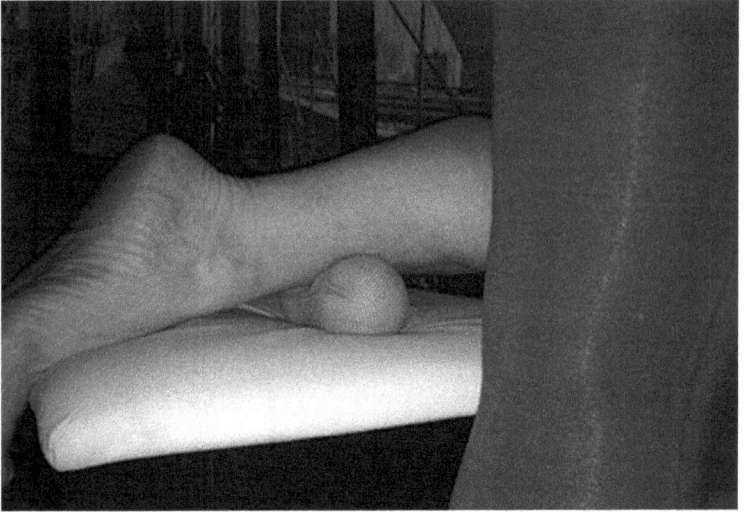

Picture 5.14: Exercise 5, step 2.

Continue to move the leg forward until the balls are in a position just above the ankle, There, reverse the movement by slowly moving the leg backwards again, until the balls are back in the starting position.

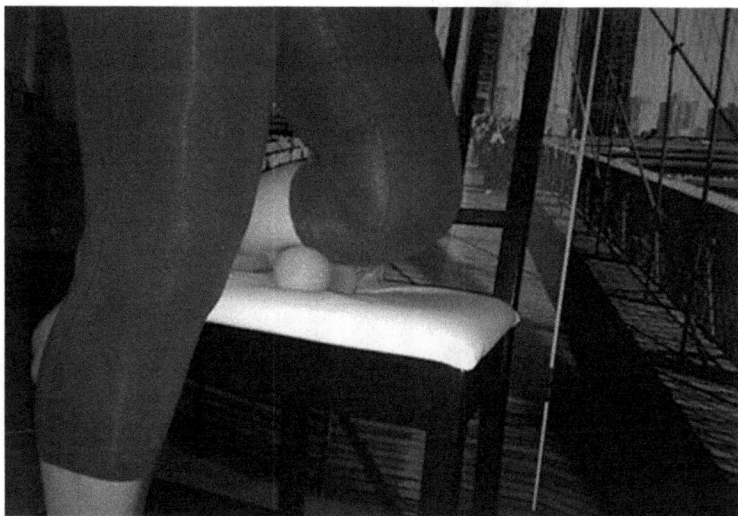
Picture 5.15: Exercise 5, step 3.

Continuously perform this movement for about 1 minute, by moving the leg back and forth. And just as before, don't rush through the movement. Try to find a rhythm that allows you to perform at least 3-4 turns. And again, remember that slower and longer is always better.

Exercise 6

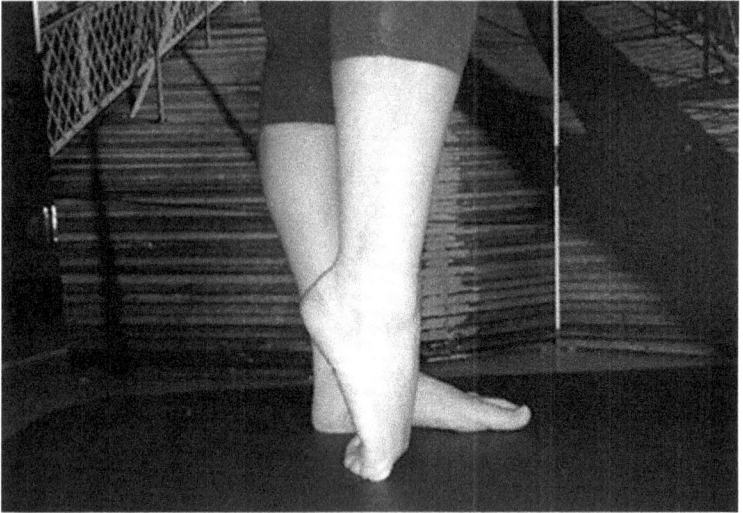

Picture 6.1: Exercise 6, variation 1.

Exercise number 6 is another stretch exercise, but this time the stretch is focused on the front of the lower leg and the foot. To stretch the muscles on the front of the lower leg and the foot, stand up with your feet approximately shoulder width apart. Next, angle the foot against the floor, so the toes fold in under the foot. If done correctly, you will feel this stretch on the upper side of the foot as well as slightly above the ankle.

Hold this stretch for about 60 seconds. Take a short break (15-30 seconds) and repeat the stretch.

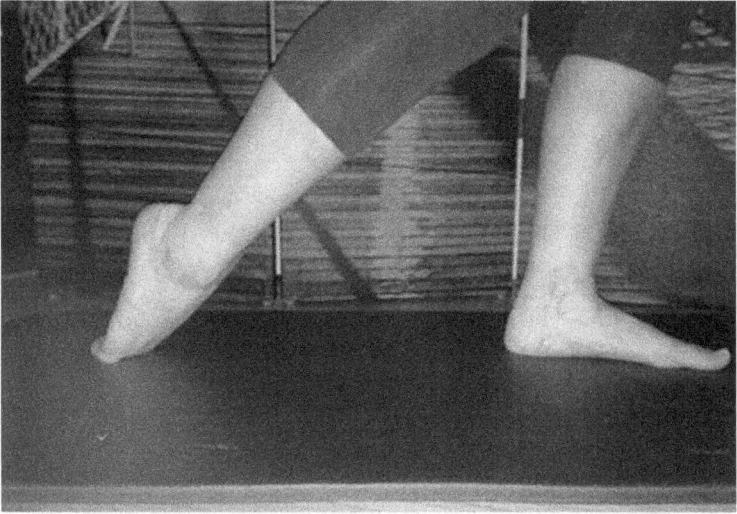

Picture 6.2: Exercise 6, variation 2.

If you don't feel this stretch in the intended areas, try this variation of the exercise, where you move the leg a little further back. Some people feel that this variation is somewhat easier to perform, so feel free to give it a try.

Exercise 7

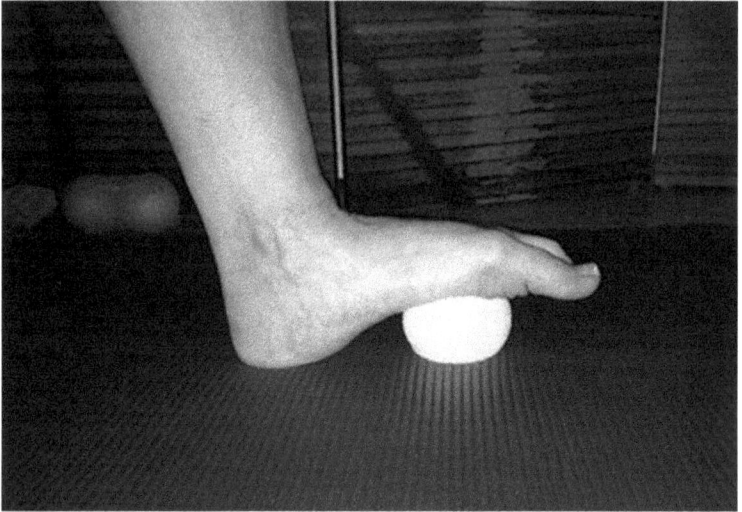

Picture 7.1: Exercise 7, step 1.

Now the time has come to move our focus directly to the foot, by kneading the tissue on the sole of the foot. Place a tennis ball below the front of the foot, as illustrated by the picture.

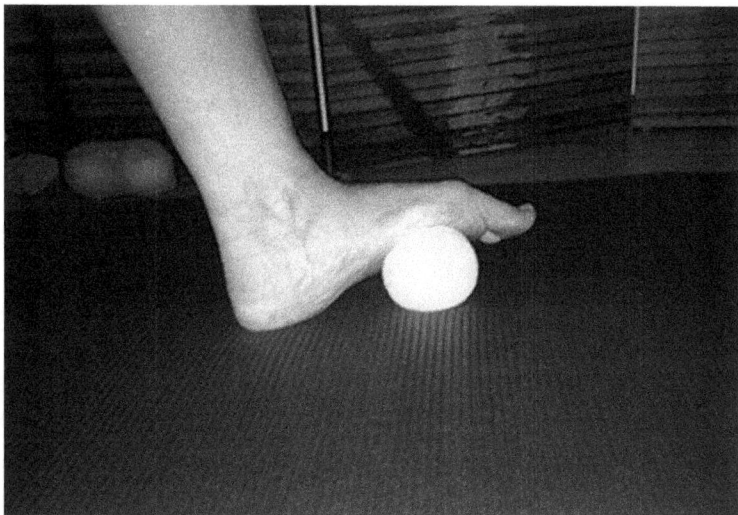

Picture 7.2: Exercise 7, step 2.

Next, "roll" the foot sideways over the ball, while maintaining adequate pressure.

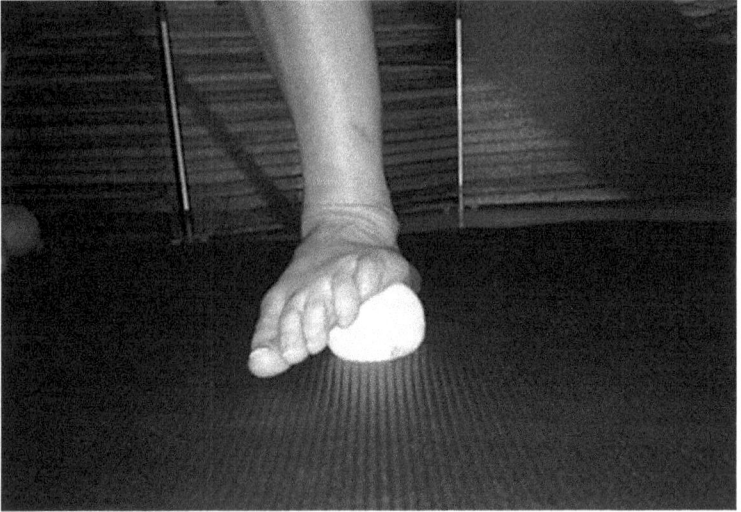

Picture 7.3: Exercise 7, step 3.

Next, slowly roll the foot back in the opposite direction, all the way to the outer side of the sole of the foot. Perform this exercise for at least 8-10 turns, back and forth.

This was the seventh and last exercise. Performing all of the exercises in sequence should take about 10-15 minutes. If adequate pressure has been applied during the exercises, your calf muscles should now feel a bit tender. However, the muscles in front of the lower leg are usually less sensitive.

6. Questions and answers

In this chapter, we will try to answer the most common questions that we have received about the program.

1. **For how long will I have to perform the exercises before I notice any improvement?**

Answer: This is very individual, and depends largely on the severity of the condition. Some notice an improvement after as little as 1-2 sessions, but in other cases, it might take up to a couple of weeks before seeing a noticeable improvement. Most important: don't give up!

2. **My Hallux Valgus-condition is quite severe. Will these exercises still work for me?**

Answer: This treatment has shown good results when it comes to pain reduction in quite severe cases. You may however need a little more time before noticing an improvement, so our advice is that you try it out for yourself.

3. **Is there any reason for me not to perform the exercises?**

Answer: If you recently have had any foot related surgery, you should wait until you are fully recovered, since this method of treatment affects different tissues in direct connection to the foot.

4. **Can I perform the exercises more often?**

Answer: Yes, you can perform the exercises every day if you want to. However, if the treated area feels very tender due to the SMR-treatment, we recommend that you take one or two days off. As the treatment continues, this kind of tenderness will usually diminish gradually.

5. When I perform the SMR-exercises, it is quite painful. Is there something I can do to lessen the pain?

Answer: Try to decrease the amount of pressure on the calf muscle by lifting the leg up somewhat, or by using softer balls. Be careful not to decrease the pressure too much, since it is essential that the muscle and the fascia is sufficiently kneaded. This requires a certain amount of pressure. As mentioned above, the pain usually diminishes gradually, so don't give up.

6. It is difficult for me to sit on the floor and perform the exercises. Is there any other way to perform the exercises?

Answer: An alternative way to perform the exercises, that doesn't require you to sit down on the floor, is to use a couple of chairs of the same height. Simply place the chairs opposite each other, with a little distance between them. Then, sit down on one of the chairs and place one leg on the other chair, on top of the tennis balls. Just remember to apply enough pressure.

7. Does this mean that I should stop using all Hallux Vallux-related orthopedic aids?

Answer: Definitely not, many of the orthopedic aids available on the market today can temporarily lessen the discomfort related to Hallux Valgus. If you feel that a certain kind of orthopedic aid – such as shoe pads or toe splints – helps you, there is no reason not to use it.

8. **I have been performing the exercises for several weeks now, but haven't noticed any improvement. Is there something I can do?**

Answer: Assuming you already apply adequate pressure, try using harder balls (like lacrosse balls), or increasing the time per set for the SMR-treatment, or increasing the frequency of the treatment (like every day, initially).

9. **I have been doing the exercises for a few weeks and have noticed great improvements. Should I stop performing the exercises now?**

Answer: Our recommendation is that you start by moving to "maintenance mode", where you decrease the number of exercise sessions to once a week. If you notice that the discomfort comes back, simply bump the number of exercise sessions per week up again. If the pain doesn't come back, try decreasing the frequency further, for example once every other week.

10. **Will my bunion diminish/disappear if I perform these exercises?**

Answer: We haven't really measured the bunions, but some people claim that the size of their bunion has diminished somewhat. For others, the discomfort has disappeared while the size of the bunion hasn't changed.

11. Can I skip the SMR-exercises and only perform the stretches (or vice versa)?

Answer: No, you can't. You need to perform both the SMR-exercises and the stretches in every session – and in the order outlined in chapter 5 – since these exercises complement each other, as described in chapter 4.

If you have any more questions or concerns, please contact us by sending an e-mail to *info@halluxvalguscure.com*. We read all incoming e-mail and do our best to answer all questions as quickly as possible.

www.ingramcontent.com/pod-product-compliance
Lightning Source LLC
Chambersburg PA
CBHW070947210326
41520CB00021B/7101